I0408390

My Journey to Independence: The Ups & Downs

By: Marcus Thadd Meyers, MSW, LSW

Marcus Thadd Meyers

ISBN-10:
154649345X
ISBN-13:
978-1546493457

Library of Congress Control Number: **TXu 2-047-053**

All characters mention in this book are real people. The stories represented in this book are true stories based on real life experiences of the author himself.

Excerpts from the following articles:
An evolution of exercise physiology: effects of functional independence with aging and physical disabilities. Roger M. Glaser
Case study on effect of household task participation on home, community, and work opportunities for a youth with multiple disabilities. Natalie Harr, Louise Dunn, and Pollie Price
Sitting risks: How harmful is too much sitting? James A. Levine, M.D., Ph.D.
Is sitting too much slowly killing you? Kayla Lewandowski
Reprinted by permission.

Editing by Rita A. Sabin, Editor I
Jacob A. Hellickson, Editor II

Front cover image printed by CreateSpace, An Amazon.com company.

Photo credit: Alex Grau
Anthony (Tony) Martin
Jarret Beck
Marcus Thadd Meyers
Brooke Gaynor
Book design by: CreateSpace, An Amazon.com company.
Printed and bound by CreateSpace Charleston, SC in the USA.

First edition printed May 2017

My Journey Independence Ups & Downs

DEDICATION

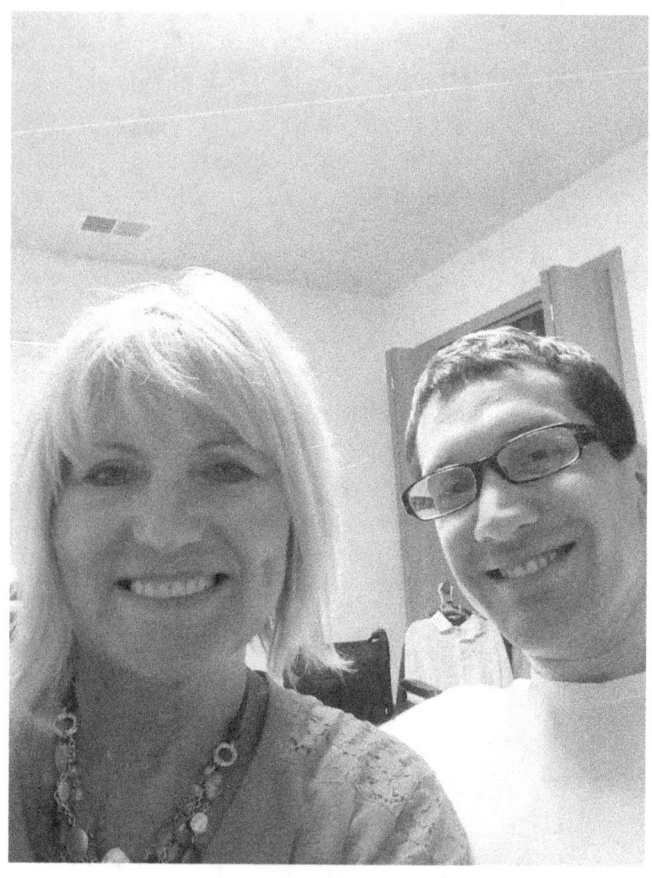

Dear Mother:

I tip my hat to you, all of the times that you have made sacrifices just so that I was comfortable! Although I was so young, I remember the days when our schedules were packed so tight with doctor's appointments and physical therapy that we would only have time for the McDonald's drive-through for a quick bite to eat. After rushing so fast to help me get to my appointment, you would help me conquer the challenge of getting on the elevators during a stage in my life when I was horrified of the elevators. No matter what, you are there for me. I remember that you and I would call hospital security to escort me and reassure me that I would be safe during the elevator ride. Although this was a small fear you did not minimize that I was scared. You took me seriously and you helped me to overcome an obstacle of riding on elevators. As I look back on these moments of fear when I was a child, I am so happy that you have helped me to overcome my elevator fear. I use elevators every day as a result of my special needs and now I am not scared.

Throughout all of my medical operations, you were there for me and you provided a comforting and healing hand when I was in pain. You stayed up all night with me being my nurse immediately after being discharged from the hospital. You were not only a cheerleader in high school, but you're my cheerleader! You helped me to persevere from the difficulties in my life related to my disability. I'm sure that you wished to have a normal soccer mom lifestyle. Rather than being on the sidelines at a sports stadium or driving me to practice in a minivan, you were there by my side at physical therapy, doctor's appointments and even by my hospital bed. This was your everyday lifestyle. Amongst all of the physicians, physical therapists and all of the other members of my support team, you are the primary foreman and construction of my journey to independence! There most definitely were a few delays along the way. You were there for me to help smooth them over.

Now that I am old enough to realize how critical it is to work hard when you are young, it has now brought me to my journey of independence. All of the pain, doctor's appointments and physical therapy appointments that I have endured throughout growing up was worth it. During times and physical therapy when I did not understand why it was so painful and why God gave me my special needs, you were there to encourage me. During times when you were the only parent because my father was away on a business obligation, you were there to encourage me! Although I have a very supportive family, they have no clue how difficult it was to have a child that grew up with a disability. Although the road is not over yet, you have definitely left a legacy that will live in my heart forever!

Love Your Son,

Marcus Thadd Meyers

CONTENTS

My Journey Independence Ups & Downs

ACKNOWLEDGMENTS

Dr. Susan Streeter Carpenter, Assistant Professor of English, Bluffton University, Bluffton Ohio

Jacqueline Ann Heil, Mother

Toledo Lucas County Public Library

Katie Schwan, Child Life Coordinator/Educator, ProMedica Toledo Hospital

Aronda Thomas, Marketing & Communications, ProMedica Health System

Lynn Closway, Public Affairs, Mayo Clinic

Rexel Rutherford, Typist

Lorie Gage Richards, PhD, OTR/L, FAHA, Editor-in-Chief, *The American Journal of Occupational Therapy,* Chair and Associate Professor, Department of Occupational and Recreational Therapies, University of Utah

Richard H. Carr, Mayor, City of Maumee, Ohio

Rita A. Sabin, Editor I

Jacob A. Hellickson, Editor II

DISCLAIMER

The author does not claim to be an expert on disabilities or cerebral palsy. If there are any questions regarding an individual with special needs performing any of the tasks listed in this book, please contact the individual's medical professional for further instructions on what functions are appropriate for the individual's specific skills and abilities.

MY MISSION

The Mission of my book is to motivate and instruct people with special needs to look beyond their own comfort zone with someone they can trust for physical and emotional support. Taking part in a fitness routine tailored to one's induvial needs can really improve one's performance and confidence level when completing daily tasks. I want my readers to gain after indulging in my book is different methods to adapt on how to overcome the challenges of everyday life. My book will focus specifically on dressing and showing and how to use adapted devices to overcome the challenges of dressing for people with special needs.

My style of writing is simply journal style with my own thoughts and honest feelings regarding the specific tasks that I was attempting to conquer at that moment. For the most part, each journal entry has its own chapter with the exception of two informational and motivational chapters.

Marcus Thadd Meyers

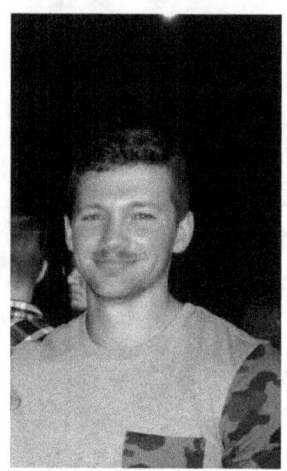

JARRET BECK

I met Jarret Beck in September 2016 at a local athletic club where he is a floor trainer. He has a certification in medical fitness and exercise physiology which provides him the opportunity to work with people that have special needs. Over our time working together, we have become great friends. I trust Jarret with my life and he will help me do whatever I want to do. There is absolutely no task that I cannot conquer without Jarret's assistance. Even when I ask for assistance, he will only give me the assistance that I need for safety reasons. I enjoy the tough love that Jarret gives me. He often uses the expression, "I just don't baby him". Jarret and I have forbidden words that we do not use during our workout time together. They are as follows: "I can't", "I won't", "I'm sorry" and "thank you". Jarret, like every other person you will meet in my book, has changed my life for the better. I am so blessed to have Jarret not only as a personal trainer, but as a friend.

Marcus Thadd Meyers

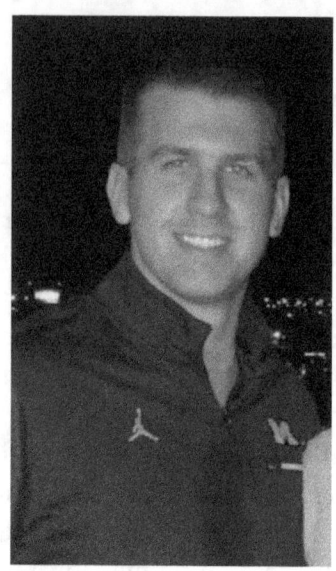

ALEX GRAU

Alex is a physically very strong man! So therefore, I feel safe with him when he challenges me to try new exercises. Like Tony, he is extremely protective. Alex also has a nickname for me and that is "Jackass". Although these nicknames may seem offensive to some, we are guys not only in this book and we all motivate each other. One of the many traits that I enjoy about Alex, like with all of the guys that workout with me, is that I am not treated like a baby or fragile. Alex has told me numerous times that he just treats me as one of the guys, as he poking me in the side and punching me all in good fun. We treat each other like brothers! Once again, I take it as a friendly supportive manner and under no circumstances derogatory in any way. As a matter of fact, Alex is a very out of the box thinker. He taught me how to put my shoes on using my sock buddy device and I am ecstatic, because it was a 100% success. Even when I felt like giving up, Alex would not let me! Alex will only help me when I ask for it, but the second I ask for it, he is right there for me always!

Marcus Thadd Meyers

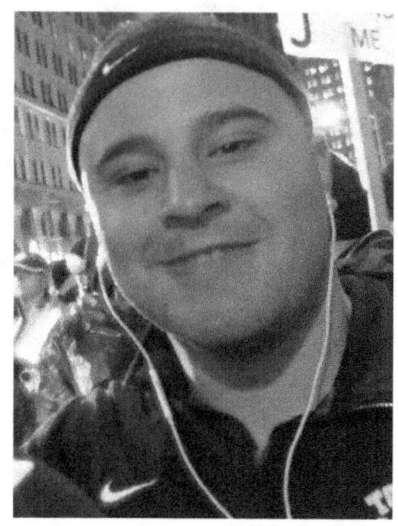

TONY (ANTHONY) MARTIN

The first phase that comes to mind immediately is "no filter at all". This makes him a stupendous work-out buddy and an extremely encouraging person, because he says what's on his mind no matter what. We have nickname for each other. If a day goes by and Tony does not call me by my nickname, I would think that he is ill. I know it may seem odd, but I do find it to be very encouraging that we are such buddies. In addition to teasing me, Tony is very protective of me and I know he would have my back no matter what, and I would have his back as well. One of his favorite ways to motivate me is to say "get going, get going", while he lies on my sofa with a pillow under his head. Tony will only help me when I ask for it, but the second I ask for it, he is right there for me, always!

CHAPTER 1

JOURNAL REFLECTIONS

The Journey has begun Saturday, February 11, 2017

Today is my first day of endeavoring to be independent, taking my own shower and getting dressed. I want to surprise Tony when he comes today to hang out with me. I dressed myself all the way except for my shoes. Perhaps it will happen another day. Note: I was putting my socks on using Sock Buddy (adaptive device) using mild baby powder, which is extremely beneficial to sliding my foot into my sock with ease.

Wednesday, February 15, 2017

Today, I talked to my friend and trainer Jarret Beck regarding leg weights. We both think that leg weights would be a good step in the right direction to help get me out of leg braces. Today, I ordered a pair of 5-pound leg weights. I am excited to see how they work out.

Friday, February 17, 2017

Today, I surprised my buddy, Alex Grau, and told him that I was able to dress myself and shower use the independently. Once again, I was a little disappointed in myself, because I was *not* able to do everything, except my shoes. However, I will not give up and I will keep trying, because I feel I am making progress each and every day.

Saturday, February 18, 2017

Today marks the end of my second week of being the new independent Marcus! I am now able to shower myself, dress myself and put on my socks, of course, with the assistance of Sock Buddy and mild baby powder. Now, if I can *only* put on my shoes. I tried that today, but it did not work out so well. Nevertheless, I will try again and I will not give up. Today I ordered a new pair of black boots online to wear without my leg braces. When my new boots come in, then I can work on putting my shoes on myself.

Friday, February 24, 2017

Wow, what a big and great week! On Wednesday, February 22, 2017, I had my one year anniversary at work. I also had my story of independence aired on all the TVs at work. If that is not enough, with the assistance of Alex Grau, I learned how to put my shoes on! I am so grateful for my friends Alex Grau, Tony Martin and Jarret Beck for helping me see past my limitations and are challenging me to be as independent as possible. Now, all that I have to learn is how to tie my shoes and that is the task for another day. It will be difficult, but I will try my best. I will not give up and I will keep going. I will get it done thanks again to Alex Grau, Tony Martin and Jarret Beck for challenging me as well as encouraging me. You all rock!

A case study done by Natalie Harr[*], Louise Dunn and Pollie Price explains the importance of allowing people with disabilities to help out around the house and with their personal care. The participants in the case study are actually the authors' own family members[*] "her [the authors'] single father and her 20-year-old brother, Jayden, who has cognitive and physical disabilities associated with spina bifida. Jayden is paraplegic and uses a manual wheelchair for mobility. He has moderate intellectual and visual perceptual defects"[2] (Harr, Dunn and Price, 2011, p. 446). The participant in the study and the author of this book share similar circumstances in regards to physical function, with the exception that the participant has spina bifida and the author has cerebral palsy.

Although this article primarily focuses on youth, the concept can be applied to anyone regardless of age. Just because the task may take more time for someone with special needs does not mean that it cannot be done. Due to the increase in the amount of time it would take for someone to complete a task, such as housecleaning, the individual with special needs may not be asked. According to research by Harr, Dunn and Price, "one reason parents might not assign household tasks to their youth with multiple disabilities is that they do not have the time required for repetition and reinforcement…."[2] (Harr, Dunn and Price, 2011, p.446).

When embarking on a journey of independence it is important that both the person with special needs and the friend or family member, agree on a realistic task to accomplish, as mentioned in *Case Study on the Effect of Household Task Participation on Home, Community, and Work Opportunities for Youth with Multiple Disabilities.* "Jayden and his father ultimately decided to address doing the dishes, as a measurable task and the father believed his son could participate in it more fully and independently" [2] (Harr, Dunn and Price, 2011, p. 447). When choosing someone to embark on a challenging task, it is important to select someone who will believe in the individual and keep encouraging them when the task at hand becomes challenging. This is a perfect glimpse into my relationship with Alex Grau. I have difficulty bending over and putting my foot into my shoe, then getting my heel into the shoe. Just like Harr "….use[d] to see the dishes at the bottom of the sink" [2] (Harr, Dunn and Price, 2011, p. 477), Alex utilized my sock buddy to help hold the shoe open so that I could slide my foot into the shoe easily by tugging on the two ropes on each side of the sock aid. When selecting a friend or family member to assist you in completing a difficult task, it is critical to select someone who has the ability to think outside the box. Alex is an out-of-the-box innovative thinker because he thought of a way to assist me in putting on my shoes. By placing sock buddy inside my shoes, pulling firmly on the foam handles and with a little upper body strength, I was able to successfully put on my shoes.

There are times when I have decreased self-esteem. During times like this, Alex gives me a pep talk and I was able to overcome obstacles just like Jayden. Friends and family play a critical part in the independence of an individual with special needs.

Sunday, February 26, 2017

Today, is my first day trying out the new 5-pound leg weights with Jarret. I used them on the treadmill because they will be a challenge to me. Overall, I enjoyed them very much and I am planning on using them by myself as much as I can.

Thursday, March 2, 2017

Today, I ordered fasteners for my new boots. I got frustrated with trying to tie my shoes so I thought for now I would just get fasteners and continue to conquer the challenge of tying my shoes. At the very least, this is a method to keep my boots securely fastened so that I can continue to go to work and be active in my community. I am so excited to put these new fasteners on my boots. This is another step towards becoming independent. For information regarding the products I used to achieve my independence, please review Chapter Two entitled "Featured Products." I will have links to all of the adapted products that I utilized to conquer the task of dressing myself.

Sunday, March 5, 2017

Today, my new fasteners arrived in my mailbox. I am so excited that I have Jarret with me to put them on my boots immediately, and I will enjoy them very much.

Tuesday, March 7, 2017

Today, I went to my podiatrist's office hoping to receive approval to be out of my leg braces. After the podiatrist watched me walk, he informed me that I have shown a lot of progress from working with Jarret Beck! If I keep working as well as I am, I can stay out of leg braces. I am so excited because after 28 years my legs can finally be free.

Saturday, March 11, 2017

Mastery

Today, marks one month of dressing myself. There are always going to be ups and downs throughout any process, but overall I feel amazing and my confidence has improved.

Sunday, March 12, 2017

Today, I have mixed feelings. I must say I had a setback due to having a blister on my foot. I was unable to utilize the treadmill and perform like I expected. However, my feelings all changed when I was able to demonstrate to Jarret how I can successfully put on and take off my shoes. He was so happy and proud of me. We smiled and joked together and that made my evening all better. I am so blessed to have Jarret as a friend.

This is a prime example of teaching your mind and muscles a new task. One's mind may be able to fully comprehend the task that needs to be completed. However, having physical special needs results in one's muscles reacting differently than expected. That is frustrating and a challenge in itself.

Saturday, March 18, 2017

Today, Tony Martin and I went shopping for a pair of exercise shoes. It was hilarious, because without my braces my feet are small. In order to find a pair of shoes that fit me, we had to go into the children's section. What a fun day we had and I loved our time together.

Exercising for an individual with special needs, can sometimes feel like standing on a stage of the biggest Broadway show. What I mean by this analogy is that an individual can feel very excited because they are out in public attempting to conquer a new task that they may not have already completed before. On the other hand, they may feel nervous or scared because people may look at them differently. They are completing a task differently than is considered normal, but still completing it to the best of their ability. Therefore, who is showing a prime example of perseverance and how people with special needs can overcome obstacles. This is just another great example of how friends can have such a positive inspirational impact, when one desires to fulfill a task that they would not dare to consider conquering by themselves.

Saturday, April 1, 2017

Greektown, Detroit, Michigan

Most of you will not understand, and I do not expect you to in any way, shape or form. It is just nice to have a group of friends that you can be yourself around. I do not feel like I was a hindrance because I needed a little bit of help up a curb, up or down a step, being pushed or having a door opened, or even being lifted off of the bus after a long, fun and action-packed day. Most important of all, I felt extremely safe and I was definitely outside of my comfort zone. It's not so much overcoming physical tasks as it is being around people who have unconditional care no matter what! I am so blessed to have friends who do not see me for my special needs! If God gave me the opportunity to change and not have special needs, I would simply say "no thank you" because of all the close relationships my special needs have allowed me to have. I do not have a disability, I have special needs and we all have special needs in our own way!

Marcus Thadd Meyers

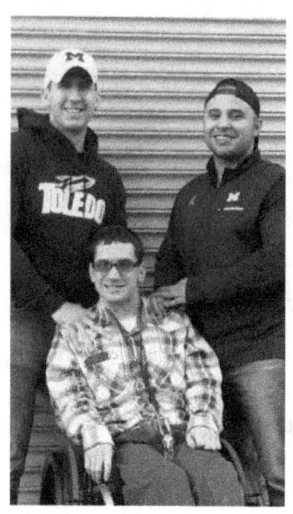

(From left to right, Alex Grau, Marcus Meyers, and Tony (Anthony) Martin. Photo Courtesy of Brooke Gaynor, 2017)

CHAPTER 2

FEATURED PRODUCTS

The is the equipment that I use to adapt the dressing process so that I am able to successfully complete critical tasks associated with daily living. Please feel free to use any of the products. I have included the links to the products so readers can find the products online.

Sock Buddy

1. Take the sock and stretch the sock over the plastic cup. TIP: Putting baby powder inside the cone will make it slide better.

2. If able, bend down and put your foot inside the plastic cup. The top of your foot is touching the top of the sock and the bottom of your foot is touching the inside plastic cone of sock buddy.

3. Use the handles to hold each side using the handle and rope. (Use the handles on each side and pull up.)

4. Your foot should slide into your sock.

After using Sock Buddy to put your sock on, you may have to reach down a little if you are able, and pull the sock up your leg. A grabber could be used to complete this action.

The Grabber

The following are instructions on how to safely utilize a grabbing or claw device:

1. Place the opened claw around the desired item to be picked up.

2. Push the trigger so that the claw tightens securely around the item.

3. Take the item to the desired location and release the trigger.

Putting on your shoes using Sock Buddy

1. Pull the tongue of the shoe back using the lace to hold the tongue. You will put the tongue over the top lace crossing. The lace crossing will now be in contact with the top of your foot. This holds the tongue in place and out of the way of your foot.

2. Put Sock Buddy inside the shoe.

3. Push Sock Buddy all the way to the back of the shoe.

4. Put your foot inside Sock Buddy; The Sock Buddy is ready for your shoe.

5. Use the handles and kick or push out hard until your foot slides into your shoe. You may have to

use a sturdy object to kick against. My suggestion would be to utilize a wall or the side of a cabinet.

- I recommend boots because they are sturdy.

Fasteners for shoes

1. There are several different types of fasteners.

2. Most of them squeeze in at the two ends of the fastener.

3. Put the laces through the fastener.

Button Pull

1. Hook the metal hook around the button and pull through the hole on the piece of clothing.

Zipper Pull

1. Hook the hook on the end of the zipper.

2. Pull the device the desired direction (up or down, left or right)

An article entitled *An Evolution of Exercise Physiology: Effects of Functional Independence with Aging and Physical Disabilities* by Roger M. Glaser, PhD, FACSM, Former Director for Rehabilitation Research and Medicine, Professor physiology and Biophysics at Wright State University School of Medicine; Senior Research Scientist at Miami Valley Hospital, Dayton, Ohio, emphasizes the ever-growing evolution of adaptive technology to conquer everyday tasks of daily living. "On the other hand, it is also essential to further develop the adaptive technology field to provide devices to accomplish ADLs [Activities of Daily Living] and societal activities with minimal muscle and energy expenditure"[1] (Glaser, 1997, p. 3). Throughout Glaser's article he makes reference to the evolution of assistive technology and adaptive devices. This piece of writing was published in 1997, 20 years since the original publication of this article. Look how much adaptive technology and adaptive devices have improved. Who knows what it will be like another 20 years from now?

CHAPTER 3

MOVE

Throughout my journey to independence, I have learned that physical fitness is critical to the success of an individual with any type of special needs to overcome obstacles and achieve their goal of independence. Completing tasks like getting themselves dressed definitely involves bending down and twisting. Do not misunderstand, it may be always somewhat of a challenge getting up and out of the Old Faithful scooter or wheelchair. Moving around in any fashion is extremely beneficial to one's health, regardless of special needs. Increased movement will definitely make it easier for an individual with or without special needs to complete daily tasks, such as getting dressed. An article by James A. Levine, M.D., Ph.D. of Mayo Clinic sates, "Too much sitting also seems to increase the risk of death from cardiovascular disease and cancer"[3] (Levine, 2015, p.1). The entire mission of my book is to encourage individuals with special needs to be more independent. For someone like myself, who is mostly wheelchair bound because of ease of ambulation compared to walking with my crutches, it is vital for me to engage in as much physical activity as possible. Everyone has a different fitness and skill level, relatively speaking, a good long walk on the treadmill is the most strenuous and skilled activity I can engage in. A study examined by Ronald C. Conner Jr., M.D., with ProMedica Physicians Cardiology, states "trying to get away from the desk a couple minutes

23

every hour can have multiple benefits"[4] (Lewandowski, 2015, p, 1). My analogy would be the human body is like a car. If the car is in a traffic jam and is idled too long, the car will stall. Therefore, the process will slow down, and the human body is very similar according to Dr. Levine, "When you sit, these processes stall — and your health risks increase. When you're standing or actively moving, you kick the processes back into action" [3] (Levine, 2015, p. 2).

Individuals who have decreased-to-no muscle function in their lower body, must rely on their upper body to complete most of, it not all of their daily tasks. Therefore, it is extremely important to maintain a strong and healthy upper body through consistent exercise. As with anyone with or without a disability, muscle function slows down with age. In this piece of writing Glaser states, "aging further contributes to the loss of functional status and creates more dependency on others performing ADLs [Activities of Daily Living] and societal activities"[1] (Glaser, 1997, p. 2). In order to best comprehend this concept, an "if, then" statement can be easily applied. If an individual does not use their muscles, then, strength will decrease. If strength decreases, then individuals with and without disabilities will not be able to complete the ADLs and other tasks as easily, if at all. As a result, they will depend on others to complete their daily tasks. Therefore, when individuals exercise they are also preserving their independence. This brings a whole new meaning to the old phrase "move it or lose it!"

CHAPTER 4

SPRINGHILL CAMPS

SpringHill Camps is a nondenominational Christian organization with overnight camps located in Seymour, Indiana and Evart, Michigan. In addition to overnight properties, churches in many different cities and states around the country also offer SpringHill day camps. SpringHill is very near and dear to my heart because I was a first-time camper there in 2000. I attended SpringHill every single summer up until 2007, when at the age of 19, I was able to become a summer staff member. I was elated when I was offered the position of Receptionist for the entire summer at SpringHill Camps Indiana. SpringHill played a major role in my independence. During the time that I was employed by SpringHill as a staff member, I was not completely independent like I am today. Therefore, I relied on my coworkers who were also my cabin mates to help me conquer the challenges of daily living for the entire summer. Having just one year of college under my belt and maturing along the way, it was very difficult for me to rely on people my own age to fulfill my daily needs. Two specific examples of the difficulties that I encountered during my first year as a staff member at camp were; having to coordinate caregivers and cabin mates so that I was able to arrive to work on time and fulfill the required expectations and I was provided a golf cart by the camp for my transportation needs around property. However. it was my responsibility to make sure that the proper maintenance was completed throughout the summer so that the golf cart would run appropriately. For example, I would have to coordinate it with my fellow cabin mates and coworkers so that the gasoline would be refilled for the following week and that other preventative maintenance tasks were completed to ensure the appropriate performance of the golf cart. I was nervous for the first few weeks of being a staff member, but after getting comfortable with my cabin mates and coworkers, I was able to communicate my needs with ease.

A large part of becoming independent is to understand that it is a process. Complete independence is not going to happen overnight. For me, it was going away to live without my parents for a period of three months, which was the entire summer. I was very used to SpringHill's operations when I was a camper, because I was a camper for a total of seven years. The difference this time was that I did not have a one-on-one counselor whose sole responsibility was to take care of my daily needs. As a staff member, it was my responsibility to make sure that I got up in the morning and appropriately and respectfully communicated my needs to the gentleman who was assisting me that day.

Although I had to take more responsibility for my own daily needs, SpringHill's philosophy for inclusion still shined like a bright star in the night sky emphasizing the fact that they let anyone who wants to come to camp come, regardless of their skills and abilities. For campers and staff alike, they provided golf carts, barrier free housing environments (without steps) and ramps for easy access. SpringHill was a very unique camping environment to me, because I was treated for who I am on the inside and not on the outside. There were several occasions throughout my summer that I had the pleasure of seeing campers genuinely enjoying themselves out of their wheelchairs and just having fun in the mainstream group, not isolated because of their special needs. The counselor would do whatever was necessary to make sure that the camper was 100% included in the activity of all the other campers. This brought me back to my camping days when my counselor went above and beyond to make sure that I had the time of my life, and I sure did!

The point of this chapter, is to reassure people with special needs that they can do anything! They may just need a little bit of assistance along the way. They may need to challenge themselves, to think outside the box, and to go outside of their comfort zone. Also, they should attempt new challenges such as a camp, or a new environment that they are not comfortable with. They may need the appropriate supports that will allow them the opportunity to discover new activities and to conquer new fears.

CHAPTER 5

WRIGHT STATE UNIVERSITY

GO RAIDERS

After I graduated from high school in 2007, I applied to Wright State University because I knew I wanted to go to college and expand my education beyond the high school level. A few weeks later, when I checked the mailbox at home, I found a certificate of acceptance along with a letter of acceptance from Wright State University's Office of Undergraduate Admissions. I had mixed feelings about this; I was both frightened and excited because I knew it was going to be a new adventure, but yet it was three hours away from my family and most of my friends.

After gathering all of the documentation from my physicians and other medical and nonmedical professionals for both physical and academic accommodations, my Aunt Ann and my Mom made the jaunt down to Wright State University in Dayton, Ohio for my appointment with the Office of Disability Services. On our way to the Office of Disability Services, I felt overwhelmed with what seemed to be a humongous campus with so many people. Once my Mom, Aunt Ann and I arrived at the Student Union, we checked in for my appointment at the Office of Disability Services. I submitted my documentation and discussed my academic accommodations with the Assistant Director of Academic Accommodations. My academic accommodations were pretty much the standard ones, which included but were not limited to:

- ✓ In class notetaker

- ✓ Reader

- ✓ Writer

- ✓ Distraction free testing environment

After discussing my academic accommodations, we then went to the Physical Assistant section of the Office of Disability Services. The Physical Assistant section of the office visit was my favorite part of the road trip, because I met B. Jean Denny who would turn out to be my friend and mentor during my explorations at Wright State University. B. Jean Denny taught a course at Wright State University that was especially designed for students with physical special needs called Managing Personal Care Assistance (ED 101).

This was by far one of my favorite courses, because it taught me every day living skills. In addition to teaching me every day living skills, it also taught me how to recruit, advertise, make a job description, hire and terminate my own personal care assistants. This was a wonderful step towards my independence. I enjoyed the class so much and I was so successful in it that I asked B. Jean Denny if I could be her teaching assistant. She not only honored my request, but she also granted me college credit for the course in addition to using me as a role model for the younger students. I feel that she helped me to focus on my strengths by allowing me to be a role model.

Marcus Thadd Meyers

During my time at Wright State University, I stayed in an accessible dormitory and apartments. The Honors Residential Complex my freshman year was by far my all-time favorite. This was top-notch because of the wonderful amenities it offered. For example, the convenience store (The C-Store), a coffee shop (The Bridge) and a small exercise facility.

When I was a student, I utilized the exercise facility located in the Student Union approximately three times a week with assistance and I really did enjoy myself. As I spent more and more time at Wright State University, I felt like I was a little fish in a big pond and just a number that no one cared about me. As a result of being so upset by the size and lack of individualized attention at Wright State University, I decided to transfer to a smaller academic institution called Bluffton University in Bluffton, Ohio. However, Bluffton University would not be ready for me to start for approximately six months. I wanted to do something fun, but it was imperative for me to stay enrolled in college.

One day, I was "rolling" by the Office of Career Services at Wright State University, when I saw an advertisement for the Disney College Program. I noticed there was an informational session coming up the next week so I went to it. To be honest, I wanted to get away from Wright State University until I could transfer to Bluffton University. That was the main reason at the time, I wanted to attend the Disney College Program. Before I knew it, it was time for the informational session. As soon as I "rolled" into the session, I could definitely tell that it was Disney due to the high energy and positive attitude portrayed by the Walt

Disney World recruiter. I too kept in the back of my mind the reason Disney was here. They were here to recruit college students for their program.

The following day after the session. I returned to the Office of Career Services to collect more information and to see how this experience could impact my college education. Come to find out, I could not receive any college credit for it because it could not be connected to my major at that the time. I still applied because I thought it would be good work experience and an outstanding resume builder.

Approximately one month later, I went to my mailbox at school and I saw a large purple folder. That moment was truly a magical one, because I knew that I had been accepted to the Walt Disney World College Program. To make a long story short, I was there from January 2010 to May 2010. During that time, I stayed at Vista Way Apartments. I was assigned to Maharajah Jungle Trek (an educational nature walk) and Flights of Wonder (a bird show) at Disney's Animal Kingdom. Participants were required to take a class during their time in the Disney College Program. The class that I selected was "Marketing You." The objective of this class was to help students to build their resumes through the avenue of mock interviews, resume writing and poster presentations. Overall, it was an honor to have Walt Disney World Resorts ® listed on my resume.

The reason why Wright State University was such a critical part of achieving independence is because it was my first college experience of living in a dormitory, and going to classes by myself. Although I transferred due to the size of

Wright State University, I am grateful for my experiences during my time there. I feel that Wright State University contributed to who I am today.

CHAPTER 6

BLUFFTON UNIVERSITY

GO BEAVERS

Bluffton University is a small Mennonite University nestled between the two cities of Lima and Findlay Ohio. With an approximate student body of only 1,400 it is very easy for faculty and staff to provide students the one-on-one attention they need in order to be successful at the collegiate level. Bluffton University may be small, but it packs an extremely powerful punch with high academic standards and with published authors as professors. Bluffton has no mercy when it comes to providing challenging courses and majors.

Not only had I transferred to a much smaller academic institution, to my surprise, I also found a caring campus community that allowed me to make friendships for a lifetime. College is not only for education; it is also important for socialization. College can be the best years of one's life with or without special needs. In addition to the smaller class sizes and smaller student body as a whole, I also enjoyed the willingness of everyone to help me with whatever I needed. I will never forget the day Mom and I sat at Bob's place (the snack bar on the campus of Bluffton University) and spoke with Jacqui Slinger for the very first time. I was accustomed to expressing my needs for accommodations to the department of disability services just like I did at Wright

State University. I was extremely comfortable expressing my academic needs because they seemed to be universal across the board. Then again, addressing personal care was the scary part, which made me uneasy. In spite of this, I persevered and opened up. To my amazement, Jacqui Slinger was so accepting of my needs she responded, "that shouldn't be a problem". As a matter of fact, she told me that she had received an email the week before of two gentlemen who would be right next door to me in my new residence hall that were eager and more than willing to help me with whatever I needed. This was such a change for me going from a big school like Wright State University, where I always felt like I had to advocate and defend every single request for services. In comparison, Bluffton was a much smaller intimate school where I never had one meal by myself. To tell the truth, there was always a group of us doing homework together. Most of the time it was in my dorm room because I had a single room whereas everyone else had a roommate. I never felt alone, isolated or like I had a special need because at Bluffton University I was not treated special. I was treated equal as everyone else. I was expected to conquer the same coursework requirements as everyone else. My accommodations were wonderful and worry free so that I could focus on learning about myself.

Bluffton University will always be a part of my life and a part of my heart forever. As funny as this may sound, a beaver was our mascot. Therefore, I am a beaver forever and I always will be! Jacqui Slinger and I are wonderful friends to this day and we will be forever! She is one of the many people that had such a positive and profound impact on my life. She was positive when I was not, she was confident when I was not, she was stern when I needed a little pep talk, but most of all she was loving and she wanted me to succeed and do the best that I could do. Thank you so much Jacqui for helping me to be the successful person I am today.

The lesson to be taken from this story is to fight back the fears and apprehensive tendencies that may come when you are attempting to express your needs to someone new for the very first time. A family member or a trusted friend can be there to support you, but it is very important that you express your needs yourself, because after all no one knows your needs better than you, not even your family. Speak up and speak for yourself even when it may seem difficult or close to impossible; you never know how the other person will respond. Jacqui Slinger was extremely accepting of my special needs and welcomed me with open arms. Little did I know Bluffton University would be one of the best experiences that I have ever had.

CHAPTER 7

THE POLICE DEPARTMENT HELPED ME TO ACHIEVE MY DREAMS

Ever since I was a small child, I wanted to be a policeman or fireman like every child at some point. Due to my special needs, I was unable to pursue that career. That all changed one day in June 2015, when I was hired as a Radio and Telephone Operator for a city near my hometown. I will never forget the day I received a call from Lieut. David H. Tullis offering me a job as a Radio and Telephone Operator. I was on cloud nine because working at a police department was my dream job. I was elated that Lieut. David H. Tullis and the police department saw past my special needs, and they were more than willing to go above and beyond to give me the best opportunity to achieve my dream job. The police department installed ramps, power doors, and accommodated me in every way possible so that I could have an equal opportunity in being successful as a Radio and Telephone Operator.

Shortly after getting the position, I looked at homes close to the police station to make an easier commute to and from work. I was thinking ahead especially during times of inclement weather. A few weeks later, I had an odd feeling of being overwhelmed and having a lot of discomfort that I was not grasping the concepts or the tasks of the position. I was slowing down other dispatchers, and feeling like I was failing my own community. On about September 2015, I talked to the Chief of Police, Jim MacDonald and Lieut. David H. Tullis, and I resigned from the police department. Honestly, it felt like a stab in the heart because I wanted to work there badly, but I felt in my heart that it was the best decision for me and my community. I would hate for someone to die because I was not fast enough to dispatch the call.

To this day, I often think about the police department and police work. I still have a passion for police work and law enforcement officers; that will be in my heart forever and never extinguished. As a matter of fact, I am currently employed at a local hospital. I feel extremely close to the security services department at the hospital because of my knowledge of law enforcement learned in the short amount of time I was at the police department. I know that when I really need assistance, hospital security will be there for me to assist in any way possible. Hospital security and my coworkers provide a good sense of teamwork and camaraderie without all the stress associated with the Radio and Telephone Operator position. Just like I feel comfortable with hospital security at work, I also feel comfortable in the community where I was a Radio and Telephone Operator. I would go there if I had a choice versus any other community, because I know they will have my back if I ever need any type of assistance.

The main intention of this chapter is to prove the point that nothing in life is a failure. Just because something did not turn out to be one's desired outcome does not mean that it was a complete failure. Everyone grows stronger from every single interaction even if we do not realize it at the time.   Thank you to the police department, Chief of Police Jim MacDonald and Lieut. David H. Tullis for helping me grow stronger as a person. I will always love and respect police work. My experience at the local police department was outstanding. Although it did not proceed as intended, it did provide me with an opportunity to achieve my dream of being a Radio and Telephone Dispatcher. Everyone has limitations; whether they want to admit it or not is up to them ultimately and no one else. During circumstances like this, it can be sometimes difficult because one has a burning desire to achieve a goal. My time at the police department helped me to realize my weaknesses so that I could turn them into positives. At times realizing one's weakness is a strength in itself, because one can bring self-awareness to areas where they need to grow.

CHAPTER 8

MAYBERRY VILLAGE

"Lights, camera, action," said the producer as the Andy Griffith Show started. That is how I feel every day that I wake up: like I am on the set of a television show. I live in an active adult community called Mayberry Village in Ohio, just outside the city I grew up in, Toledo. It is truly a replica of the village in the show. Complete with a clock tower, Floyd's Barber Shop and Andy and Barney's bar and grill right in our little village. I thought that would be an ideal time to mention that at one point there was even a police substation in the village. There is even a car show which takes place primarily during the summer months. Mayberry Village plays a significant role in my independence because it is here that I live in my first apartment by myself. The apartment is fully accessible with one bedroom and one bathroom while fitting my needs perfectly. I am the youngest resident in the community and sometimes as I pass by other residents, I hear them say, "here comes our young whippersnapper." I would like to make it very clear that Mayberry Village is not an assisted living facility, but rather a 55 and older fully accessible community. The reason why I am permitted to live here is because of accessibility reasons, all apartments are on the ground level. I can transfer easily from wheelchair to shower because it is flush with the floor and there is a handrail near the toilet, so that I can easily keep my balance. Communities that market themselves as a 55 and

39

older facilities are permitted to have a small number of residents that are under the age of 55, while still being classified as a facility for 55-and- older.

The reason why this chapter is critical to my book is because it illustrates that people with special needs do not have to be institutionalized or live with their families all of their lives. If their desire is to live on their own they can, as long as they are able to do so safely.

CHAPTER 9

INSPIRATIONAL QUOTES

The intention of this chapter is to help boost motivation and energy during the "down" days of your journey.

I have learned that anyone, regardless of their skills and abilities, can do whatever they put their focus on. They just may need a little push of assistance.

Attitude is everything; If you think you can do a task, then you can. If you think you cannot, then you cannot.

Go outside your comfort zone; do something that you may not think you can do. For example, go to visit or join a gym. You may need to go with someone that you trust if you feel you need that type of support.

Do NOT compare yourself to anyone else; Always try your hardest in all that you do. One hundred percent is 100% for everyone; the number does not change based on physical abilities.

Dedication (wanting to do something consistently) + innovation (finding new ways to conquer a task if the standard way is not feasible) = success (task completion)

LINKS FOR FEATURED PRODUCTS

Sock Buddy

https://www.amazon.com/Sock-Foam-Grip-Pack-Blue/dp/B01ITXUIAG/ref=sr_1_1?s=hpc&ie=UTF8&qid=1489455932&sr=1-1-spons&keywords=sock+aid&psc=1

Fasteners

https://www.amazon.com/gp/product/B00GYSB3HG/ref=oh_aui_detailpage_o00_s00?ie=UTF8&psc=1

https://www.amazon.com/gp/product/B014X6MM70/ref=oh_aui_detailpage_o01_s00?ie=UTF8&psc=1

Grabber

https://www.amazon.com/gp/product/B0002VUQPG/ref=oh_aui_detailpage_o02_s00?ie=UTF8&psc=1

Button & Zipper Pull

https://www.amazon.com/Ribbed-Handle-Zipper-Pull-Button/dp/B009R2LNSA/ref=sr_1_6_s_it?s=hpc&ie=UTF8&qid=1489584492&sr=1-6&keywords=Button+aid

REFERENCES

Glaser, R. M. (1997). *An evolution of exercise physiology: effects of functional independence with aging and physical disabilities.* Journal of Rehabilitation Research and Development, 34(3), vi-viii.

Harr, N., Dunn, L., & Price, P. (2011). *Case study on effect of household task participation on home, community, and work opportunities for a youth with multiple disabilities.* (Reading, Mass.), 39(4), 445-453. doi:10.3233/WOR-2011-1194

Levine, J. A., & Mayo Clinic. (2015, September 04). Sitting risks: *How harmful is too much sitting?* Retrieved March 15, 2017, from http://www.mayoclinic.org/healthy-lifestyle/adult-health/expert-answers/sitting/faq-20058005

Lewandowski, K. & ProMedica Health Connect (2015, June 22). Is Sitting Too Much Slowly Killing You? Retrieved March 14, 2017, from https://promedicahealthconnect.org/wellness/is-sitting-too-much-slowly-killing-you/

FOOTNOTES AND COPYRIGHT PERMISSION

[1]From Medline "An evolution of exercise physiology: effects of exercise on functional independence with aging and physical disabilities," by Glaser, R. M., 1997, Journal Of Rehabilitation Research and Development, vi-viii., p. vi-viii. Copyright 1997 by this content is in the Public Domain. Reprinted with permission.

[2]From Medline "Case study on effect of household task participation on home, community, and work opportunities for a youth with multiple disabilities", by Harr, N., Dunn, L., & Price, P., 2011, (Reading, Mass.), 39(4), 445-453. doi:10.3233/WOR-2011-1194. Copyright 2011 by IOS Press and the authors. Reprinted with permission.

[3]From Mayo Clinic "Sitting risks: How harmful is too much sitting?" by Levine, J. A, 2015 (http://www.mayoclinic.org/healthy-lifestyle/adult-health/expert-answers/sitting/faq-20058005). Copyright 1998-2017 Mayo Foundation for Medical Education and Research (MFMER). Reprinted with permission.

[4]From ProMedica Health Connect "Is Sitting Too Much Slowly Killing You?" by Lewandowski, K. Copyright 2017 ProMedica and ProMedica Health Connect. Reprinted with permission.

*Family member of researcher

Marcus Thadd Meyers

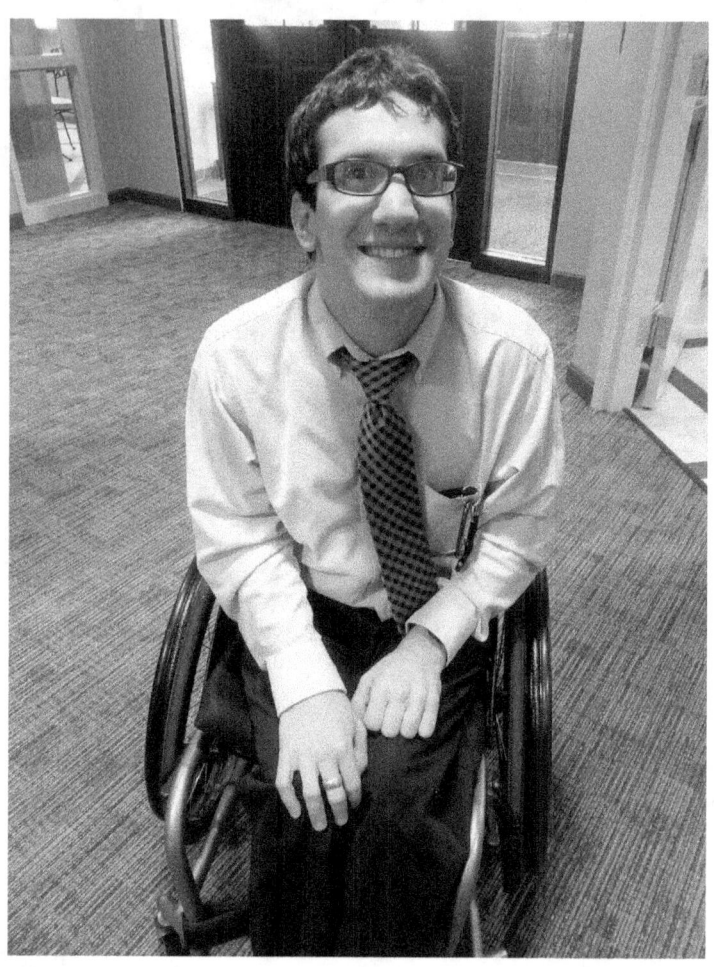

ABOUT THE AUTHOR - INTRODUCTION

My name is Marcus Meyers. I graduated in August 2012 from Bluffton University in Bluffton, Ohio, with a Bachelors of Arts in Social Work. After achieving my Bachelors, I went on to challenge myself by attaining my Master's degree in Social Work at The University of Toledo, in Toledo, Ohio. The field of Social Work has always been close to my heart because I have some physical special needs that has allowed the pleasure of interacting with licensed social workers frequently. As a matter of fact, I feel that Social Workers have contributed to my success today as a well-educated independent adult. Ever since I was old enough to understand the meaning and functions of Social Work, I wanted to pursue this profession. I felt this was my way to give back to what was given to me. Even though I have overcome a great number of obstacles in my younger years, it was not until my mid to late 20's that I really did realize that I am starting to overcome the physical obstacles directly related to my physical special needs. Buckle up and enjoy the journey to independence. It is common to assume that my family has been a great impact on my independence. However, that is not always true. Do not get me wrong, my family continues to support me and still has a tremendous impact, but for me the greatest amount of support was my friends. I am most inspired by people close to my age. Throughout this journey, you will get to meet all three of them. There will be some setbacks throughout the journey, but please tighten your seat belt and press on because that is what I do each and every day.